ALKEDEMA

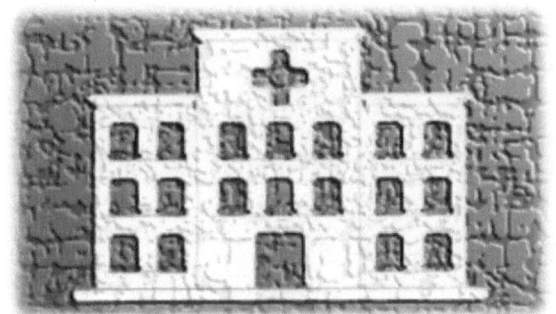

Field of Blood

By

ALEXANBDRA SONSON

Table of Contents

BIOGRAPHY

Trying to get a sense of my profile, I drew out portrait of the exile. It has been awhile since, I mapped out Canada as Sugar Land. My life is as sticky as sugar cane jam in my hands. My name has not change since then. I bare sticky ink on my hand from a runny pen. I am Alexandra Sonson, still the same girl from the island. I once reside among friends and rodents. I have got one great listener and lover; He is the Only Son. The first piece on this paper is dedicated to Him. My voice has been in silent mode. I am not out to be rude. I never intrude. I am not here to pry. So, would you listen to my cry?

"In this world all are hustlers – forced to bow down to the rich man's alter"

Alexandra Sonson

DEATH INSTITUTE

Locations of Satanic Operations

The subject of the anti-Christ is common knowledge, and so common that he is raining on our parade frequently wherever we go. The reality of Truth as presented to me by Jesus Christ is this; one cannot detect the anti-Christ just by analysis and characterizations. What are we hoping to find? And where are we looking?

The have cultivate a culture of death amongst our people that is projected and presented as the new future. Because of the concentration of evil in our midst, many are consecrating themselves to the prince of this word rather than to the Prince of Peace. As a result, people have no peace because we are constantly fighting illnesses, diseases, enemies, poverty, and plagues. The scripture clearly confirms it in this passage.

My people are destroyed for lack of knowledge: because thou has rejected knowledge, I will also reject thee, that thou shall be no priest to me: seeing thou hast forgotten the law of thy God, I will also forget thy children Hosea 4:6.
The most undeniable fact is the reality of how much the world are entrenched in new age teachings. Sadly, through all these practices,

we are ignorantly dragged into witchcraft. We practically give wizards, warlocks, sorcerers, murderers, access to our homes and our physical temples so that they can explore and exploit our beings at nights. Then they drain our entire system out.

Jesus has given us the answers to these underlying concerns. Since Jesus has given me warning over and over in Ezekiel what ramifications are at hand to those of us sent and to bring the gospel to nations but choose to withhold information, I promised to leave no stone unturned. This world is so theatrical in nature that it spreads a blindfold on those of us who has conformed to human standards. The blended system that we adjusted our senses to has turned us all into commoners. Because of the dramatizations on televisions and other forms of communication networks, we all get entangled in their nets.

Satan is sitting on the throne of our living room. Satan sits on the throne of our souls. Satan sits on the throne of our congregations. Satan sits on the throne of our minds. He just sits because his members are seated there also. In this context, this text will sharpen; awaken something so that we can all adjust our minds if you may. The main and major topic here is to address and highlight individual territories and methods of operations as prescribed by Jesus Christ. Living can be difficult for a true believer of God. As a chosen vessel of God, to act as an Ambassador is to get a glimpse of hell on earth, and to experience the wrath of the Destroyer accordingly. Living for God comes with many challenges because the angel of death sends his followers to come and wage war to remove the seal of God over your life. What you see and who you see are not what they portray themselves to be. What the enemy wants is to thrust a man of God into doubt and uncertainty. Satan works with high influential being with ranks and power. The prideful agendas of every man are to build a reputation and to have his or her image immortalized behind a glass case.

Everyone may well know that members of organizations are rallying for Satan and it would not matter one bit to me if Christians and I were not their dart board for targets. Right now, let us forget about the hunters and go straight for the kill.

THE ART OF IDOLATERS

Death on the Rise

Jesus, once more deeply moved, came to the tomb. It was a cave with a stone laid across the entrance. Take away the stone, he said. But, Lord, said Martha, the sister of the dead man," by this time there is a bad odor, for he has been there four days. Then Jesus said, did I not tell you that if you believe, you will see the glory of God?" So, they took away the stone. Then Jesus look up and said, "Father, I thank you that you have heard my prayer. I knew that you always hear me, but I said this for the benefit of the people standing, that they may believe that you sent me."

War has been has known to have brought the most causality in history. Living apart from war most people believe that life was peaceful and safe. Most information was filtered through census and mouth to mouth reports. Now death in a country, nation, city, or town has toppled the figures brought about by wars. People are dying faster through manufactured diseases, and sickness. Everything that was once classified as genetic makeup or genetic inherited diseases are a bunch of fabricated lies. Everything society has used to explain certain sicknesses and diseases are manufactured, thus making everything taught as false. There is only a two-way street about information, it is either true or false, no middle ground.

It is necessary to put a name and a face to Medical Institutions to provide a more accurate details to an audience about the subject that is on display.   The exploration of medical department gives you a display and insight of its operation both inside and outside of its domain or bounds. With intent to drive a spear through the heart of the framework and format of systemic operation in the medical field, we will examine the **Philology, Etymology** and **Terminology, Psychological, Anthropology, Theological, Spiritual, Sociological** aspects of these properties.

The **etymology** of language is not a field commonly studied or practiced by many. Satan is clever, and the people that work his department are cutting and shrewd. Have you ever noticed that when an authority figure, an elite person example a physician comes with a diagnosis, he or she present information before a subject without expertise in that field or area, then they use some grand **terminology** to explain the situation? And that person, not having any background in **Philology** answers what?
Then they bring the big words down a notch, but you still leave that department in a fog. You are given an answer that half satisfies your

concern. Whenever, you encounter a situation in the medical field, it not your two cents they require to proceed with the procedure, but rather an agreement. Most people voluntarily agree to things they know not. Let us look at an insurance enrollment for a change. When a telemarketing sales representative call a person's home to sell you an insurance, they will read out the marketing script without mercy. The customer never understands a word from the list of information provided. Once upon a time, they would throw in a bonus a watch or something else and finalizing the script that it is all for free. But there was a snare in all that beautiful presentation, a cancellation period that most of the buyers forget to do before the four- or six-weeks period, then they get charge.

Nothing has changed except that telemarketing and robbery has grown to a new level through technology. It is outrageous that a person can use someone else name to make grand purchase and burn tires driving glamourous vehicles robbing another person. It has been made known to me very clearly through the Holy Spirit the degree of blindfolds that blocks the vision of nations, territories, and countries. The call is not to throw darts at one nation or a people but rather to address world curriculums. I do not care about building a repertoire, this whole project that JESUS called me to record is so that He, God can put an end to the ruthless butchers that slaughter lives of human beings.

The play on words is operating as a mass grave. On the **Psychological** plane, many people give their lives away just by signing a contract. Many, many things in Canada requires the signing of a contract. Signing a lease contract is signing a deaf certificate. If a man is lucky enough, they might escape through the system unscratched. In previous manner, I have explained how my landlord patronized my life, but now I will go further to explain how the Lord dispatched me to the bedside of my niece on the verge of dying on a hospital bed. Developing a habit of preparing a **Doxology**, worshipping, and acknowledging God's goodness is extraordinarily rewarding. Our God is Almighty, and our God is worthy to be praised. To God be the Glory.

Scientist have expanded the branches of Science hoping to find ways to equate human development with the foundations laid down in Scriptural laws, decrees, statutes, and the commands of God. The competition is gliding its way through the system in a very sly and devious manner. Example the branch of **Anthropology** covers a variety of teachings. The nature behind all this investigation is to be able to set a table of extended branches that can bring us a lifetime of study so that we are unable to discover the mysteries. The main reason behind these studies to explore and exploit mankind genetic dispositions is to bring further confusion. The confusion is not about who we are but discover how to eradicate and terminate life. People are already being terminated based on medical historical backgrounds. If a person comes with a certain ethnic background and a climate with a strong history of cancer or other diseases, science develop a method to continue and prolong the agony of death in such areas. To a scientist, a person's medical background determines the size of the label he or she is carrying. And many sicknesses are developed over time through secret operations performed by another human being hired from the dark side.

Biblically speaking, the study of **Theology** is a study of life. The word of God is the breath of God and learning and practicing the life of God to extend life. When the Bible is taught by lecturers, it is not in a way that it should release the Holy Spirit or the breath of God. When the Holy Spirit begins to educate a man, it comes like a trickling of a faucet and them it begins to rain, it begins to pour, and it becomes inevitable for the mind to dismiss. The sound of the Holy Spirit galvanized His presence like rain drops falling on a metal sheet. When Jesus gives that silent knock on our hearts, the sound gets louder and louder until there is a two-way communication that dispel all doubts. And it is no longer Jesus who seeks me to deposit life in me, but I in turn seek Him for more. Many men and women do not understand the power of the Word of God, because they do not have the Spirt of God with them.

The language term **Spiritual** is extremely broad and carries several meanings. Whereas, to some people, it is simply a religion. Religion is a topic that many people do not discuss, and by avoiding the subject, we are paving a broad way as broad as the term leads. In my case where I was living as an open book and one many people gladly open and shut and left on a shelf deserted, it was through deep rejection that life's challenge took me to the highest plane in my life. Sometimes, we ought to go back and thank that person(s) that frankly and heartlessly rebuked and buffeted our flesh.

I once held a lot of displeasure and anger for such a treatment. But the height to which I met JESUS CHRIST is incomprehensible, inexplicable, the exuberance and the love of Christ comes in my state of unrest. I am so overwhelm with Joy in the LORD, yet my heart bleeds from afflictions and wounds of wicked hands of tyrants.
Sociologically, I experience a dis-connection to friends and people overall. Absolutely everything in my life suffered. I went to work walking under a cloud and came back to a

place where darker sheet spread over my horizon. I have not been able to keep my emotions in check for an exceptionally long time. However, there are days and moments where I will wail and after wards, I will laugh uncontrollable. We cannot tell what the Holy Spirit is doing or feeling sometimes.

The lord asked that I pray for soldiers, as I sit in the corner of my room hiding like a soldier eating a bowl of instant noodle soup on a Sunday, thinking of the soldiers positions of danger, I realized that I cannot even compare myself to one. But an overwhelming feeling of sadness and an un-controllable emotion burst out of me, I began to cry. I could not stop the flow of praying in tongues as I weep.

GOD'S INTERVENTION

Justice for forsaken and the forgotten

Son of man I have broken the arm of Pharaoh king of Egypt. It has not be bound up to be healed or put in a splint so that it may become strong enough to hold a sword. Therefor this is what the Sovereign Lord says: I am against pharaoh King of Egypt. I will break both his arms, the good arm as well as the broken one and make the sword fall from his hand. I will disperse the Egyptians among the nations and scatter them through the countries. I will strengthen the arms of the king of Babylon and put my sword in his hands., but I will break the arms of pharaoh and he will groan before him like a mortally wounded man Ezekiel 30:21-24.

Enchanters stand far off in the galaxy to perform acts of wickedness, provoking children of God. They have stood long and strong perpetuating mystical beliefs. They have stood hidden in crevices of rocks driving arrows, bows, bullets penetrating hearts of innocent souls. Evil doers have greatly advance transporting primitive customs and practices. These wicked people have gain powerful roots robbing individuals dreams, visions, and aspirations to advance the kingdom of hell.

People that operate in the kingdom of darkness come stealing finances, shooting men down with invisible arrow, bows, bullet and even using their vehicles to run you over. Idolaters carry a permanent mask, while they present themselves with charisma and full of spunk. They all have double identity. They appear normal and natural human being by day. And they are criminals by night. However, one who engages in idolatry, have split genes. Their hidden profession as hit men and women is performed openly without anyone knowing their perpetual wickedness. We are dealing with criminals, wicked people, murderers, and thieves. And they can stand boldly and protest. They can use a good rebuttal you know. All my family members that workers of iniquity have monopolized and butchered, it will be accounted for. Those that once had my life on their chest board and shifting hands to knock me off the board will seek no more, they shall find me no more, they shall gamble with my life no more.

I have been watching enchanters in action working as ushers throughout this COVID19 but, JESUS IS LORD OH! They seem to think that they are in control, especially the malice in their eyes when mine locks into theirs.

What gives them that power for them to want to think that they are giants and we are ants to be crushed under their feet? Their strength is in their high professions and titles. Through systemic rejection and discrimination, they use all types of techniques and rebuttals to bring about injustices. They had gotten away with robbing me; and rubbing me the wrong way for way to long. You see, every time I fought with one, I would take the matter to our Heavenly court. Each time, I would address it with God and leave it thinking that He will never answer, and that the wicked would keep making weaklings out of us. Never did I imagine that all the tears shed was being accumulated in heaven for this time. We watch the wicked prosper and continue to exercise power on the children of God. Let the scripture be a lesson for the wicked.

God does not delight in the strength of a horse, nor his pleasure in the legs of a man…Psalm 147:10.

I have seen wickedness, and I have seen the wicked in action beyond compare. All the evil performed on me to stop my calling, only God can repair. At some point in the trial, I wail so hard and without a doubt it was a call for revenge. These merciless human beings left me restless and, in such agony, I could not even stay focus on the Lord. Now, I have finally given in to God completely and I am calmer in the storm.

The fellow shoot me down by using my poop as a missile against me, but after two and a half years of not using the washroom, I do not know where he got the poop. But May 6, 2020, he shot poop at me again. Unlike other times when I rant and rave, I said nothing. The following day, I recorded it and put it up on social media. The next day, he tried to keep a low profile. According to my Heavenly Father, when you do not hear much from his side, he bottled up praying, and I can hear the silent stamping because he is a noticeably big fellow. For the devil to have his children harass a child of God to that extent is beyond comprehension.

Whenever the stench was released in my apartment, and whenever I am in the bathtub, I would blow my hornet. I examined the situation and I would say to myself this is not the works of a human being. It is a situation that God has promised to take care of but never in my wildest imagination that I would anticipate such inhumane activities. With everything the Lord kept unfolding before my eyes, reading the scripture had me crying, raging, and I promised God that I would not back down and that every work of the devil would be exposed until the very end. And I will not go back on my words. Those who do not understand evil suggest that I move. All though they practically knew now thing about the situation, just the fact that I must use the washroom off site. Unless God solve this problem, there is no escaping. God is not the son of man that He should lie, nor a son of man that He should repent of His sin. I AM WHO I AM says the LORD.

My commitment to God has grown stronger with each passing moment. When these people came to scatter my life and frighten the day light out of me so that I would not see the day light to persist and continue what Christ was doing in me, they almost had me begging for mercy. The one thing they did not know, and underestimate was the power of the King of Mercy that was operating inside of me. Still they had me running from one end of the spectrum to the next. I run from the North to the South, they followed. I run from the East to the West, they followed. I run to the United Sates, they followed. To top it off, one of their men tried to refuse me entry into the United Sates without any valid reason. For that matter, I told him that I was attending a Christian conference program. But they already knew my purpose, and this is exactly why they fought me so hard.

THE AWAKENING
Breath of God

The scripture tells us that, "The LORD reveals Himself to those who diligently seek Him". One of the early signs and characteristics given to me in my youth was the ability to have accurate dreams and my spirit was able to detect, feel and know what another person was thinking about me. However, I dismissed all these signs out of ignorance. I cannot say that I knew God then, but I spoke to him then and call upon him. There was a part of me that knew that He is the All-knowing God. Whenever I experienced injustice, I always go to God first, and even sometimes after cursing those who cursed me. If you asked me, I would tell you now, I did not know any better and I did not know God either. I knew about Him very well if that counts. When I got called, I would have visions of my exam paper beforehand, and I never knew what it was until after the exam. I adopted a habit of writing down things but got extraordinarily little time to go back and review what I wrote.

The beginning of the battle, everything in my life and my family's life were declining. But the pivotal event in all of this is when I received a text to tell me that my niece was hospitalized. I was told to wait for further news, when the news came back the text indicated that she was in ICU. That was just another term to add to my directory of acronyms. I had just booked a flight to go to the USA on a conference., so I had time to visit the ICU right before I left for America. When I got to the ICU, my niece was in a comma and it did not even matter whether I had gone without seeing her because she did not know that I sat at her bedside for about an hour or more before I left. I started asking the nurses questions and how long will she be hospitalized. The answer I got was an exceptionally long time. The day before I left, I went back once more time. I realized that the atmosphere had changed, and I was under observation. I prayed over her and anointed her with healing oil, but a hospital staff happen to come back right on time to witness the anointing taking place.

Whenever a person is under the influence of the Holy Ghost and you hear the Holy Spirit voice get moving. The Lord asked me to go back to the hospital immediately when I get back, and I did just that. I visited the hospital the next day, and I got there right on time to find her missing. The same nurses saw me came in but none of them said nothing. I went back outside thinking that I had entered the wrong room. And I must admit that the person they said that would take a long time to recover was out of the coma. They had transported her to another room.

When I began visiting in the other room, I arrived right on time to find emergency workers strapping her on a stretcher, because she was being transferred to another hospital. It was then that the Holy Spirit put me on high alert. And I did not know why but still I was trying to find employment, but I had difficulty with my work email password, so when the email asking me to report for work came through, I never got the email. When we live to rely on our own feeling and emotions to feed our hunger and desire, we do seize to understand and corporate with the Omniscient God.

Throughout my wrestling with my thought, I blindly walk in the move of God to visit at the hospital. I frequent the hospital, and the idolaters kept a logbook about my arrival and front desk would quickly alert the nurses that I have arrived. They thought that their activities were a secret.

An increasingly great sense of desperation to quickly kill my niece and do away with her was rising. Because God knows the human heart and everything, He made known to me what is written in the governmental laws and societal departments and systemic flaws that swift through. So, I constantly stayed at my niece's bedside. During the period I am at her side, she seems to be improving. But whenever I leave for the night and return next day, she is in decline.

By the Mercy of God, the Lord began to speak to me about and against that territory. Whenever the LORD brough me to a point or location, it seems to appear that I appear in the area by default. For God everything is planned and programed in heaven. There is a connection to everything that takes place in our country and society. God has lay out and iron out everything through these series and things taking place for centuries.

Final message to people who are adding to the kingdom of darkness is that God's mercy and judgement is here, and it seems we are at a stage where much finger pointing is taking place. There is a reality beyond what is measured by human flesh, and beliefs. As I God called me forth out of recklessness, I have reached a point from restlessness to restfulness.

Let the LORD be magnified and let the scripture cause ripples in your stomach. Therefore, this is what the Sovereign Lord says: *In my wrath I will unleash a violent wind, and in my anger hailstones and torrents of rain will fall with destructive fury. I will tear down the walls you have covered with whitewash and will level it to the ground so that its foundation will be laid bare. When it falls, you will be destroyed in it; and you will know that I am the LORD. So, I will pour out my wrath against the wall and against those who cover it with whitewash. I will say to you, the wall is gone and so are those who whitewash it, those prophets of Israel who prophesied to Jerusalem and saw visions of peace for her when there was no, declares the Sovereign LORD Ezekiel 13:13.*

.

LIFE AND DEATH
The Weak and the Strong

The medical arena is at the tip of the pyramid
and it is most influential and significant for
promoting health and human development.
People both great and small seek to find
solace lying on a hospital bed. Understand
that God is the author of life. And the scripture
tells us that Satan is the author of death. Many
people ignore and dispel the idea that Satan
exist as myths rather than believing that He is
actively working in our midst.

Hospitals are time zones, and there is an
agenda. Realize that there is a chart on every
patient's wall with a history of that individual.
Realize also that a man's medical history has
been designed as the outlet that determines
whether one live or whether a man die.
Realize that there is generational pattern of a
history of the type of death that clouds a family.
Realize that the hospitality that meet and greet
us has become more and more sophisticated.
The physician no longer asked questions,
rather a patient is welcome by supposedly a
nurse that enters the room with a chart and
records. They will question the intended patient
and asked to further screen your process while
walking the line of Divinity.

There is an ultimatum on our lives, and it is written in hell that certain human being may not pass or meet a certain age.

Satan's judgement is passed through the very system that screen, scan, photocopy, and collect information about our lives. We were made to believe that the system is to serve and protect our identification, instead our information is being used to duplicate, replicate, imitate our lives. The devil's judicators are passing judgment left to right back and forth. They are found in the North, in the South, in the East and in the West., occupying jurisdiction, and passing out judgments. Our God is **Omniscient God**. He is the All-Knowing God. Our God is an **Omnipotent** God. He can do all things. Our God is an **Omnipresent** God. He is everywhere at the same time. Unlike the Almighty God, Satan strives on anticipation. God do not need no chaperone. He acts alone.

Exploring what drives the medical department and how it is operated is an extremely dangerous ground to tread, but I will go there because JESUS sent me and it involves me, my family and future family members. When the wicked decided that they would make an example of my family member, they fail to realize that they cannot take God out of the equation.

When the wicked kept me in the back burner and only to turn up the heat higher and higher, I called even more to a Higher Power. When we think that God is not listening, yet still believe in Him enough to address our problems to him and hand over the plaintiffs or our prosecutors to God, the matter is set before him whether we want to believe it or not. God do not care about how well you know Him or how much prayer we put before Him. As He made known to me and reminded me that His Father is a lawyer. God was telling me that He is taking care of it. Did I ever anticipated that God's hand would be so powerful on this mortal and sinful body? Oh! My God is God, He makes the law, He passes the judgement, He declares who is innocent or guilty. He makes the ultimate judgement; He is the ultimate judge.

I come to testify today, not to be concern about what another man thinks. It does not matter who believe, or who reject what I have to say. Hey! I am no lawyer. I am not even an intellectual, and I have chosen not to wear such robe. Especially after seeing through the garment of reality what it entails. I say what God tells me to say. I do what God tells me to do. I reveal only what God wants me to reveal. And I can only apologize to God if I acted in error and put forth some of His information out before the appointed time. On the other hand, our God can override any error.

Working simply with heavenly help was not easy. It was the greatest comfort knowing that the strongest and best team was on my side. Frankly, I was looking for a God of Moses to do some damage while I witness it to talk and write about it. God does not really operate as He once did during Moses time. The Lord is feeling a lot of grief over the attitude of no believers.

While I have grown to muster strength, I will honestly say I have grown more than anything. The confession that I must make is this, only JESUS can endure the degree of abuse I experienced on my body. Many of the things that people experience as demons are manually performed by wizards. The fellow is using a method to break my system down. The Lord has provided the acronyms. However, I believe I need to explain what the Lord is doing in bringing me to a clearer understanding.

That man monitors me so much inside, and I know it is not through any demon. Whenever I go to the fridge, he is at it working on my head stamping to trigger my mind. Whenever I stepped into the washroom, he is coming to, he runs ahead of me and open the water. But apart from all this terrorizing and tormenting, he has a companion below helping him out. Whenever I seat down on my bed, the fellow below me sits. And he has some type of devise fighting and poking and penetrating my but. He is using some form of spatula whisking something inside of me. My intestine and stomach have become their cooking pot. Then the fellow above me is working in synchronicity with him. Do you know guys, they have not stop fighting to destroy me, even though they know that I have recorded all the methods of wickedness by which they operate?

So, if these guys are operating in a home with limited resources killing people every day. How much more are the ones in the hospitals are achieving? LORD, only you LORD can bring me out of this without hatred. It drains me emotionally and physically knowing a landlord collects government money to kill tenants. And the hospital in turn gets paid for every patient that is admitted for brain injuries. People, everything is a connection as the LORD reveals to me. It is almost like there is no way out. One of the things that has been bugging me since beginning is the rising of condominiums. The City of Toronto is literally kicking people out of homes to build condo. Guess what, the operations are even more grandeur and greater in number. The bible gives so much warning about the shedding of blood through witchcraft.

God is bringing serious judgement on planet earth. It scares me, and sometimes in my wailing, part of me is afraid that the righteous will perish along with the wicked. God's wrath is burning, and it will not quench until everyone returns. And I tell you, Idolaters are stubborn. They are raising all types of riots; we are dealing with under cover rebels. The rebellion we are experiencing during the COVID19 is no secret to me. I know that my God is working for our good. All the high-profile criminals that stood boldly and fired me and rehired me because of this work needs to repent. All those that attempted to fire me and come back thinking that they can sign a treaty with me to get me back must reconsider.

You see, these men and women doctors and nurses putting patients under serious anesthetic or sedatives to help them weaver away quickly will account for their actions.

GENETIC MAKEUP OR SATANIC SETUP
God is Fed-up

When the ark of the LORD had been in Philistine territory seven months, the Philistines called for the priests and the diviners and said, "What shall we do with the ark of the LORD? Tell us how we should send it back to its place."

On Friday April 17, 2020, in a vision, Jesus said: "My Father, on this earth there is no value. It is time for me to see the difference, no value, no value, and then He began crying". Then, I arose out of the vision and recorded it. In May 28, 2020, I had another vision of seven angels dressed in white blowing their horns.

The kingdom of God is crying out against the kingdom of darkness. The kingdom of darkness know that it cannot penetrate the Kingdom of Light so, they are crying out wolf! wolf! wolf! when there is no wolf. The only thing that they work with is time and waging nasty wars to cause delays. What we do not understand is that the fight takes place in the spirt realm, and in the physical realm they come to open doors to stagnate one's plans and visions. But God sees them waiting and watching for their prey under that tree, at the three crossroads or in front of a rock. While another man may not be aware of their activities to be vigilant, these vigilantes keep vigil day and night until they have caught their prey. Many foods that were life saving for people that lived in poverty survived on has been known to kill. But it is not the food that kills man, instead a man that operates in the dark realm is sent to kill another man's soul leading to death.

Occultisms is so intelligently designed that it acts like a vaccine or vacuum. Many, many Christians are drawn into that system, and we even sit on their board of directors to assist in doing modification and application to improve and advance the system. We contribute in the planning and redesigning of methods and means to refine that body. The extremely high secret society diviners operate upon is not exposed to reality.

The revelations that the LORD, Jesus Christ has revealed to me is disheartening but is the reality of the dark scroll that God must unfold. Medical institutions are held in high regards because it possesses the history to resuscitate lives and assist in bringing new lives into this world. In what the kingdom of darkness performs and seeks to gain, God light permeates and pierce through the darkness.

The hospital is their domain because it is a time zone for death. And the second hospital where my niece had been admitted is an inferno. It is because the territory is inhabited

by an Indian Muslim community. I went to Tim
Hortons and asked for a tea after being
neglected for some time. I made the purchase
and went back to the ward. The Indian girl
gave me coffee. It was a deliberate move; I
took it back and said to her I asked you a tea,
but you gave me coffee. Her friend
apologized. The reason why I was so adamant
about letting a sick patient drink that coffee is
because, the wizards at my apartment had
mixed something in my coffee jar at home.
 She took it to change and brought it back and
said you said that you did not want it too hot,
would you like me to add some ice cubes?
This really confirmed that the coffee was
deliberate. I answered no thanks, took the tea;
thank her and left.

The very moment I entered this hospital,
attempts to ambush me is being made from all
walks of life. From the staff to patients, and
visitors. Usually, I leave the hospital late at
nights and arrive home about 11PM. While I
am preparing dinner, I am being shot at by
those in my apartment, the one below and the
one above. The court case with the landlord
has only intensified the matter.

July 7, 2019, it is evident that no matter where I
go or what I do, or do not do, trouble troubles
me. I sat at the bedside watching Veronica
recovering at the hospital. She likes to use the
hand that is working to touch things, besides

the nurse told her that she must exercise the hand that is operational. And one thing she does is to pull on the curtain that divides her with the other young girl beside her. Besides that, the curtain is the only thing accessible. There were two other young women visiting the girl and one just suddenly got up pulled the curtain away from Veronica. I said, she does not know what she is doing. She snapped and said, "I don't care." I reminded her, "this is a hospital." She answered, "that's right, I shut the hospital blind." I said to her, well that is just mean and that is evil. It is the just and the unjust right? She went silent but she had just stirred my juices. She angered me so much I wanted to go on and on. It is about the upper class and the lower class, the rich and the poor, the blue collar and the white collar, and the elite against a nobody right! I wanted to tell her Oh! Miss Universe should have her own private jet, and her own island with her own hospital. And by the way; you are a bully. But when I opened my mouth, the Holy Spirit stopped me. I just laugh and said Jesus, Jesus, Jesus.

Visiting hospitals and deaths were becoming common, and I do not wish to become an acquaintance. The first main attack happened with my sister's spouse. Only with the help of God that an analysis of his death rings true in this matter that I am compelled to address. Joseph lived in a government apartment during the time of his death. Looking back and drawing out sketches of his symptoms, I can make a clear cut and complete analysis of his symptoms. Joseph suffered the exact urinary and bowel movement problems that I experienced before God showed me what was destroying my life. Having said that, I am also compelled to mention that my friend and my friend's friend living in government housings are under similar attacks. Therefore, can anyone imagine how many more people has died or are dying from the same attack by idol worshippers?

Joseph was having loose bowel moments and his entire system cave in. He became sluggish and was wobbling and struggling to maintain his balance, and he was slurring his speech. He died a brutal and ruthless death. He had just left the hospital that day after a long hospitalization stay. When he got to his apartment, he fell on a center table, split his head open and bled to death without anyone by his side to help him. My sister was at work at that moment. It was pass the hour when she got off work and found his lifeless body.

In my case, it did not get to the point of a doctor's diagnosis because of the Great Physician in Heaven, JESUS. It was through this same vicious attack that revelations and the revealing of the kingdom of darkness was made bare by JESUS. When I speak of systems systemic flaws, an examination and an analysis of the operations provides proof of how families, peoples, nations, and others are perishing through witchcraft attacks. Because a landlord had decided upon my fate by positioning a felon or a fellow upstairs above my unit to assassinate me, the LORD wrath was kindled against the wicked. That man was poisoning me using hydraulic system and chlorofluorocarbon gradually poisoning my inside. Had I not been a prophetess in the spirit realm and the Holy Spirit was not giving me information, he would have made a dead man out of me. The Lord knows the works of the enemy long before it is orchestrated. The enemy always go with intent for mass destruction that will leave casualties, casualties everywhere. If God do not have your back enemies will stand strong. It should never be so, therefore; I cannot emphasize enough that knowing the word of God is a lifesaving jacket and knowing our God parachutes us upward in straight velocity. Otherwise all we are is a small astronaut with a spacecraft/rocket-ship waiting in obit.

After the wicked murdered Jefferson, they went after my sister and drove her away unto the Streets. A perfectly sane woman just started to be stalked and haunted by demons. I had to witness the shift in a life of someone I love where she went from sane to acting insane. By the way, she was a powerhouse and the first to ever give her life to Christ. She went to the Holy Land and came back and made a serious prophecy. She mentioned that the Canadian dollar would be stronger than the American dollar. It happened immediately afterward, and it was then her life drastically declined.

Then soon it was my father that died. Then my sister in law got hit by the same dark experienced that catapulted her normal working life, leading to a brain aneurism and two strokes that soon cause her death. That death was not an accident either, just another common act. The mask the wicked has been wearing is the same, and they have been clowning around, so no one is able to identify their faces. Almost a year later, another sister back in Saint Lucia got attacked and suddenly died. The Lord revealed to me that she was under witchcraft control and it was confirmed. They work with time; they work with cycle and follow a certain pattern. Now my niece is under attack with the same brain aneurism that led to two strokes. When she came out of the coma, she said to me they said that they came for me. I asked them what have I to do with you? They said that they want my whole family.

July 10, 2019, as I got off the hospital elevator, there was a group of about 12 people standing at a counter. I recognize them all to be east Indians. They were conjuring evil spirit inside the hospital while praying for another hospitalized fellow. The hospital guess rules are two guests per patient. Yet, in some rooms will have more than what is stipulated, and they can gather in large groups such as these.

LORD unto us O'LORD, LORD unto us. It is Biblically outlined that the commander of darkness is the creator of sicknesses and diseases, and the author of death. He is not staying just in the hospital you know! He dominates and terminate lives through system operations. The hospital by far is his number one domain where his practitioners achieve his commands on massive scales. Before I can walk readers through, a few encounters with death and the hospital, the demonstrations and illustration put on paper will be able to tell the story better than anyone.

I am on a rally for Jesus. July 23rd, 2019, I arrived at the hospital earlier than usual. When I entered the hospital ward, I found Veronica slumped down over a tray of food almost untouched. It felt like I had just entered a shipwreck with an unconscious passenger still at the dining table, and everyone else had escaped. I went into a frenzy and asked for the nurse assigned to Veronica. The woman that claim to be the nurse quickly answered after I asked whether anyone ever assist Veronica with her meals. I was furious and told them, that I have observed several unethical instances where Veronica is singled out and neglected. I had been taking notes and recording and tape recording. After I took a stance, the atmosphere changed and became very serene and serious. I spoke of previous day's when I sat in the room and for two and a half hours straight as I tried to find Veronica's nurse to change her diaper. These nurses are all pretending to be highly in demand and overbooked while they waste much time debating and chatting in the hallways.

None of them are aware that I am tape recording as well as journaling. There are moments when Veronica was making great progress. There are days when I arrive there unexpectedly and she is in delirium, drugged, and chasing away demons. Her speech is more slurring than anything else. They do not even give a sip of water. I asked for a cup of water for her many days ago. Twice she had adhere to my command and drank a few sips. Otherwise, the cup of water is just there. The week of July, the Lord finally made me realized that what the enemy started from a person's establishment, the hospital staffs are located to finish off the unfinished business. The development and demolishment are so subtle, it goes on detected for centuries. Coming to the hospital and getting immediately fired up only make them sound the alarm louder to alert the other members. Already, there is a watch tower raised up for me at T.G.H. Before, when she was at S.B., no body tried to fight back, they just kept on the lookout and quickly transferred her.

At T.G.H., the numbers of idolaters are vast. They have members shooting at me. Their monitoring devices are constantly turning at the four quadrants to detect me. There was a time when I tried to reason with myself asking, how do they know I am coming in? Now I know without a doubt how they program things starting from your dreams, then to the mirror you use, the coffee you drink, the water you use, your residential place, the alarm system, the person that owns buildings, the area that you live, friends you associate with and the list goes on.

In the beginning of my Divine Calling, I received all the warnings in the spirit realm and kept asking myself why I was being watched in black vans, motorcycles, and all other types of automobiles. My so-called career tricked me and kept me busy like a squirrel seeking peanuts to try and stay alive. The enemy thought they had me then. They sent plagues in the place to scatter me but the fighter that I am overthrow them when the Lord showed me that it was an attack. They began to throw other tactics. The battle ensued.

Since then, my Divine Calling sprang forth. My thoughts can never be man's thoughts. I am programmed by JESUS CHRIST you know. When I arrived, Veronica was sleeping and going in and out. The nurse came and changed her. Afterwards she began to talk to me saying I have had enough of the Osler family. I do not know who they are. She went on telling other stuff that did not make sense. Then she said, so many people, they came to get me. I asked them what they want with me. They said they want my whole family, and they want to make them all crazy. That was a confirmation of what the Lord revealed to me on May 28th. A whole year later, the Lord revealed that she was referring to the hospital and staff.

In this series, trespasses through the medical territory for man to understand the grounds upon which we stand, the documented sources present a documentary for viewers. Journeying through the same passage multiple times, death once seemed to be a natural path. Death plagued my family so often that, we became immunized by the sting from the syringe of death. We all accept death as an inevitable fate regardless our faith and belief. It is only through the Mercy of God that road once travelled ends. This treacherous journey could be insurmountable if no one takes account to represent the family or this generation of Christians. Everyone wants to take a new spin, a new perspective on life. Our mindsets are centrally located to focus on things around us, and we do not go beyond our jurisdiction.

The hospital is a place under Satan's dominion. Before I can walk readers through, a few encounters with death and the hospital, my story lines are enhanced allowing me to be able to tell the story better than anyone. Living in the silence of indifferences may have its ancient ring. Living in Cult City, and in a country where witchcraft is religion is beyond understanding and a man of the flesh will not grasp. The painful darts are not mere sting coming from wasps. It is a detestable story to tell. Images spread out on pages are raw, gruesome, and grotesque. I am grudgingly trying to grapple the grisly attacks from ruthless monsters. They maul the flesh like sharp molars of a shark's bite. Only, if only one could see the fangs raging out of their close jaws. They are pretenders.

It has been a harrowing and horrifying situation. Sometimes, I would be awaken by the slumber, thinking in retrospect, looking back at the years I have not been able to stand under a shower and let the water jot my memory down is downright depressing. Standing inside a bathtub and pouring water over my body with a cup reminds me of a baby who is afraid of getting wet. But as I stood back and watched the prophecy of Ezekiel unfolds, and manifested in me is astounding and unbelievably believable. Everything the Lord asked of Ezekiel has happened to me by the book. The reminder that I try to maintain is that, we do not wrestle with flesh and blood but against principalities (principals). You see, the hospital gets paid for every patient that comes in with a brain aneurism, but it has left me wondering whether the income doubled if the operation result into a person's death.

GOD'S JUDGEMENT FOR BLOOD SHED

The word of the LORD came to me: Son of man, will you judge her? Will you judge this city of bloodshed? Then confront her with her detestable practices and say: This is what the sovereign Lord says: You city that brings on herself doom by shedding blood in her midst and defiles herself by making idols, you have become guilty because of the blood you have shed and have become defile by the idols you have made. You have brought your days to a close, and the end of your years has come. Therefore, I will make you an object of scorn to the nations and a laughingstock to the countries Ezekiel 22:2.

Nothing is hidden from God and no crime is left unpunished. The people of the dark kingdom know that better than anyone else. It is in knowing that they fought to fill my mind and my body with filth both during the day and at nights. People that are performing wickedness never expect their deeds to catch up with them. They have navigated their way so smoothly and for so long that to them it is inevitable that someone else would find out.

Witchcraft operations has spike the labor industries and causing it to boom. While they rising to reach the height of heaven, someone else's life fluctuates, spirals in down word motion. Technology has open means for them to dodge and swerve their way right through to stardom. And in that same manner, the shedding of blood has grown because of the internet. It involves the shedding of animal blood, human blood, or any type of blood that qualifies and satisfies for a sacrifice. Since the LORD laid down the laws, commands, decrees, statutes concerning shedding blood, God will not make adjustment to the law, and His laws will not change. The ten commandment is written on a stone tablet for mankind to abide with and for all generations. The Stone tablet represent the Living Rock who is JESUS, who come to redeem all mankind.

Everyone knows that going against the Living God's law is demonic. The only people that will find my work offensive is those who operate in opposition to what the laws say contradicting TRUTH.

STENCH OF DEATH
End of Hospitalization

When my niece was sent home, it was said by doctors that she would never recover. Not knowing that in the early stage of her hospitalization, preparation had been waiting approval to pull the plug. Everything under writers' prescribers, doctors, and specialists, I override it with the word of God. Jesus is the greatest physician and He has been on my side.

After Veronica was released from the hospital, Jesus brought me face to face with the incomprehensible to make life more comprehensible. My niece was also under demonic influence and attack like I am. When the hospital ambulance staff carried her in on a stretcher, that very moment, the devil was working and preparing for a grave accident. The stairs leading to the basement is very narrow, and the people carrying her asked her to keep her hands in but evidently, she could not and perhaps did not even understand a word. In trying to make her keep her arms on top of her stomach, the fellow holding the back of the stretcher kept shouting causing a commotion leading to confusion and the poor girl holding the stretcher fell inside and almost broke her leg and almost drop Veronica in the process.

The minute I got at my niece's home; the Lord immediately led me to discover that she was under the identical attack that I am facing. And to make the evidence even stronger, the fellow had the same name with the monster above me. He introduced himself as Saul. In like manner, the one above me introduced himself as Paul. It was not a coincidence, what the Lord led me to understand is in fact, the names these monsters hold are given or taken according to their strength they presume to possess. They are dealing with water, water spirits if one may say. The thing the Lord drew me toward one day is Paul's journey in the storm on the sea. Afterwards a serpentine spirit had latched itself unto him. But Paul just shook that devil out. Acts 27-13-14.

The landlord excitedly came down to make his appearance. Perhaps in his mind, he thought that he could finish my niece off along with me. This was a battle I nowhere where near anticipated. While the hospital was silently drugging Veronica to slowly kill her, I was battling legions of demonic entities and people. But when I took the task to care for her, it was a gamble with my mental and physical abilities. The monsters living above her as husband and wife, Oh! I tell you, I am lost for words, and I do not even have words to describe what I went through. The monstrosity, the degree by which evil prevails, and evil doers live and breed among us is an injustice and it should not be taken lightly. A normal people do not have a clue about the depth and the type of disaster they bring about on mankind.

As soon as Veronica return home from the hospital, Oh! Man, what a trip, what a journey. What monsters who stood in the way to make us trip and fall. Monsters that just wants to push the wheel of death to keep the cycle flowing. And that fellow began to come and get his laundry done every Sunday hoping to finish off his victim. I knew that she never did anything to that fellow who wants her dead because I never did anything to mine either. Still I investigated, and asked questions. The answer I got was that, Veronica started to have severe headache when she moved into this home and doctors diagnosed it as migraine headaches.

However, when I got to her apartment, the fellow Saul started paying me visits, and immediately began to open doors for me too. I rebelled against him and fight the system like a Ninja. Whenever they know that you know, they will start to drive their tractor trailer or to bamboozled you and throw you off the curb. So, he fought, I fought, he fought, and I began to fight even harder. As I come to allow JESUS to use me to screw in the nut bolts of darkness, let it never be loosen again. They come to strike like lightening bolts, and they come terrifying victims like thunder bolts. Let them strike their heads upon the Living Rock when they come against me. No matter how much they entered my apartment to curse every possession I owned, even releasing curses on a small basket with my dry goods and can foods inside, my God is alive. No matter how hard they curse, JESUS can only be curse once and it was so that this day, he can take away my curse as promised.

During Veronica's recovery state, demonic operations working above her head was rapid. The attacks on her mind by the husband and wife was mind blowing. It was so severe; the forces of darkness were hoping that I would give up and collapse. When her situation put my life to a halt, adversaries at public places, institutions, and around her home magnified. Unemployment denied me and drained my capacity, credit card debts escalated, and all the calculated strategies of the devil raised my level of anxiety. I had not reach a point of anger in months, and anger raised like a flame of a burning raging fire. When help was needed, no one lifted a finger except for her stepfather, my brother and sister that provided money to her sister to buy food and diapers, as necessary.

September 4, 2019, the day was a bit frustrating. I had begun to meditate on the situation rather than the solution. It was beginning to look like a mountain. I knew in my heart that the Lord require that I do this but without financial help and I had an apartment to maintain with my things in it, the impediments in my finances were blind siding me. Oh! How I had become gasoline for the devil's fire. While the fellows in my apartment attempted to physically break my spine, government institutions continued with the maneuver and manipulations emotionally to make me more susceptible for breakage.

At Veronica's apartment, the fellow has a huge boiler room right next to her bedroom raging. That same boiler room is where the laundry machines are kept. It made his victims easy target to have access to the laundry room too, and every weekend at that. In that same boiler room, there is what assumed to be a storage room with a lock on it. My nephew says that is where he keeps his winter tire. But every devil worshipper keeps an altar where they feed evil with blood or whatever. And the fellow has access to that room. They are so cleverly organized that the sink inside the laundry room has a huge suction hole that swallows socks, under wears and other things. When I began to feel other evil manipulations taking place in my body, the answer came back when he suddenly returned one side of my sock and placed it on the side of the sink. I never noticed it missing either.

THE DEVILISH BUCKET

A storage vessel

A concept or theme about filling buckets to keep one's overflowing is a common thread that runs through multiple systems and methods. One of the common threads that runs in institutions is the ability to steal through public access and outlets. Robbing another man is so easy for idol worshippers that they do not sit and think about it, they just perform because they can. Performance is what their father the devil requires. They just generate huge double daily quota to resound in hell.

These wicked idolaters are generating evil based on the principles of the Bible. They expected to continue to swerve their way through this system and this planet without ever having to be accountable or even being discovered. What they did not know is that God waits for an appointed time.

The wicked keep time so that they are not caught in the act of committing that crime, robbery, murder, or whatever they are out to perform. They keep track of the children of God every second to know what the best time is to loot and invade lives. The skillfulness, their prominence, and their great exploits will not be remembered, nor is it acceptable in the kingdom of God. Or need I forget that they are laboring for the kingdom of their father the devil.

Behold, the nations are as a drop of a bucket, and are counted as the small dust of the balance: behold he takes up the isles as fine dust. Isaiah 40:15 kjv. You see, every bucket they have filled without God giving them permission will be taken away when ever that bucket drop.

The spirit of God within me noticed and revolted against everything that these idolaters were doing with the help of children. These adults only had to see me for them to begin some form of retaliation against me. They look at my size and my condition and saw me as so vulnerable and ignorant, that they can just sit at their throne and violate and mutilate my thoughts and body without me knowing or feeling a thing. At the end of a day's work, I would be conversing with JESUS and crying buckets of tears.

The thing that was the hardest to grapple is the attack in my unit thirst thing in the morning before I left for work. The stench the fellow boldly used to prepare the way for me before is the most unfavorable and memorable image difficult to let go. When one examines idol worshippers who are out to get you, they always pretend to be on the scene by default.

While filling bucket is time consumed, it is so significant for them to maintain. Whenever, I show up in a room, the wicked adult would raise the subject to the young ones about replenishing and keeping their buckets full. They are all aware that God is about to strip them of what has been stolen to return it back to His children through me. Many of the things that they tried to keep hidden from me was carried out in codes. The things that the LORD would reveal just blows my mind away at times. At times, my emotions were so confuse and delicate that JESUS would have me laughing so hard, they would just give me that stern look in anger.

God was just laughing at the wicked sometimes. Some of the things that finally felt amusing were just too painful to revisit. Without the spirit of God, I would just bask in anguish and with hatred. There were times when I just let things go and tell them just what I think of them. The flesh does not have tolerance for evil deeds and arrogance. When I found myself glued to a hospital bed, with no income and fighting further systemic injustices, the deprivation left me with even a greater sense of desire to crush the heads of systemic injustices in Canada. Fighting the same battle year after year and month upon months had grown too familiar and too frequent. The devil's children have had the handle of things for so long that in their mind and in their hearts that their secrets would never be unearth and that they can be never be disarmed. Further down in that same scripture, we see how the enemy works through deception when Rebekah cause Jacob to steal Esau', his own brother's blessings. What this illustrates is a degree of covetousness, envy, and jealousy and a lack of concern and love thereof. The craft in witchcraft have been in practice and is operational since Biblical times.

The line of covetousness continued to stretch in Genesis between Rachel and Leah.

THE WALL OF DELAY

Precursor of Time

The devil does not know what God is doing, and the only thing the enemy does is to lay claim on a man or woman of God by stalking him or her around. You see, when I tell someone the degree by which my life is miserable with such people, they respond with doubt. I do not think that too many people know the type of blatant missiles that are fired at them daily. Each time Satanist cause a delay they pitch a fork in the way, or they dig a staff in the ground to halt another person.

 Imagine, these day light criminals will leave a string of dental floss lying on the step waiting for me. Do you know what the dental floss is for? They must operate in the physical to go right down to business in the spiritual realm while you are sleeping. They want to destroy the structure of my teeth in my mouth to be able to delay the deliverance of this message presented here today. They had two green alcohol bottles on an altar using to turn me into an alcoholic. When I brought it down in the realm of the spirit the bottles became useless. They left them lying on the garbage bin the next day. They are running out of ammunition;

they have tried addiction to sweets exposing me a chocolate bar on the step in the doorway.

The compulsion and obsession of members of the dark ages to turn me away from performing and from doing the will of God makes me turn away from them with repulsion. The seduction and the way in which the enemy pry and come to make a prey of an individual, they are like dogs sucking liquid in a suction cup. Have not they come to realized that JESUS do not come finding people with a hook or bait. JESUS just stands on water or sits by the well. Whenever you hear people use the word wickedness, I do not think that too many people understand what it really means. We have a people that maintains a profession that requires killing people, destroying lives, tearing down another man's establishment without reason simply because they covet other people's possessions. They are jealous of other people lifestyles and they come with an agenda from hell to snatch and loot what belongs to someone else.

GRASS ROOT MEDICINE

Precaution is better than cure was the concept people lived by. Medicine used to be a simple cup of bush tea, no preservatives, no combinations, no portions, with just an added scoop of sugar. People died natural deaths except the occasional hit and run by white and black magicians. People often knew when a person got hit and they would go around in the village whispering and gossiping for they knew who the actual witches and warlocks were in that vicinity. We heard these secrets about enchanters and took note of it. People were told that a witch caring an incantation walked on the left of the intended victim and they will never pass any other place except on your left. Even if there is not any more space on the sidewalk, they will climb the hill just to remain on the left side. As children we would run to the other side of the street to make space for them. Anything people warned parents about was to keep their children away from such people because they like to roll their hands on a child's head in circular motion. That simple gesture was a sign that they were stealing the child's memory and virtue. Parents knew these things, and they refused to allow anyone else to rub their children's head.

We touched another decade and another period when things began to change, and that means people were forced to leave their young ones in daycares, schools, babysitters, and other means of caretaking. People are living in a vulnerable stage, and vulnerability leads to disability. The first thing I noticed when I came to Canada in 1900's was the rate of disability. When the Lord drew me out of my comfort zone to educate me about a system that failed me in every way, that call is one that shed light on a nation and a people to reveal the skillful aim and schemes of wicked foes. When I drew a portrait of the whole systems' systemic flaws that kills a society secretly, silently, smoothly, and rapidly, it is to say to potential victims beware and take note.

The discovery brought to me by God's grace point to me that I was living in a house where I was being manipulated by magicians came in a very unexpected manner. When the Lord called me forth, I kept having visions and dreams that I was under observation, and that I was being monitored. I kept looking for a camera installed in the wall or something. I found none so I continued to move around vicariously but my mind refused to dismiss the matter. So suddenly, the Lord asked me to cover my mirrors, that time I listened to the voice of the Holy Spirit and covered the mirrors. There were also some very strange activities taking place also with things just falling off without it being touched. This one I dismissed as a natural phenomenon because I had extremely limited space and thing were piled on top of each other.

The parts of the room where a person spends the most time during an ordinary day has been marked and secretly designated for witchcraft activities to take place. First, an outline of the manipulatives, schemes, vices, and devises have been mentioned. I will attempt to give a better explanation and provide a better understanding of the situation involving the hospitalization of my niece who experienced near death with a brain aneurism. Prior to my niece diagnosis and trials that God walked me through, it is also necessary to mention that my brother's wife died with the exact brain aneurism. In that very same vein, I was the one that spent the most time at her hospital bedside because everyone else worked on a very rigid and strict schedule.

Then suddenly, one day while sitting on the hospital chair, I had a vision of my niece with a teddy bear under her head. The Lord started to spike my mind with ideas, so I began to investigate, asking around whether she has a teddy bear on her bed. Then I was told yes. When her sister and I arranged to go and clean her apartment before she leaves the hospital for her home, we wanted to make sure that that teddy bear had gotten rid of. When the investigation started to peak, it was after I was forced to move in with her because she still did not have comprehension, she still could not walk or stand, and she was in a total paraplegic state.

I have become like an investigator; I went about asking her son who is situated above her and I even went about asking for background information about those living above her. What type of people are they? The minute she came back, the man started to quickly frequent the basement, doing weekly laundry. The first thing he did, one day was to quickly go at her side and tried to talk to her. He needed close contact to work on her further. I was not happy, I had to tell him that she does not have comprehension yet and she does not walk either. But that was not news to them, Satanist keep a track record.

The track record or medical record a doctor or hospital keeps is to know how long the line of generation and the line of longevity in that family is. They also need to know what type of sicknesses or diseases run in that family in other to lengthen the history of that sickness or create a new one. Satanists is not as smooth as they appear to be.

When my sister in law got hit with brain aneurism, she had no blood connection with us, just the same last name because she carried my brother's last name. Suddenly, brain aneurism would begin to dominate the family line and use as a genetic transportation or transmutation. The saddest part of it all was the other person who suffered that same brain aneurism beside her was a Christian. When I sat at Veronica's bedside, the patient beside her had visitors. Two Muslim women came to visit and when they thought that I might suspect them, they walked away saying God bless. When I told her daughter that she had visitors and who they were, she was puzzled and said that they are probably women in our building.

The LORD gave me the encounter with the monster above my head in which I fought a wicked war because the man was operating profusely and endlessly on my mind. It was so that I could have hard core evidence, and that no stone would be left unturned. The LORD brought all these wicked activities to light so that this brain aneurism would be just a passing phase in history.

While the girl was in hospital, the staff that had been station to finish her off were working diligently and deliberately. When evening I came out of the elevator floor to visit my niece, a group of about twelve workers of iniquity were conjuring up demons in so called prayer mode at the front desk area. It was after their juju did not work that they decided to let my niece go home for they realized that they could not get rid of me and they needed to preserve the reputation of the hospital and staff.

Disability and sickness are manufactured in homes and apartments by workers of iniquity. While a person is fast asleep without even saying a prayer, these robbers are pulling their triggers. They beat a silent drum all night and every hour. They do not sleep, for any Christian who is out there and not engaging in even saying the OUR FATHER, Satanist is sure to keep a logbook and they are parading on your head throughout the night. What Christians fail to realize is the busy operation of night watchers whispering lullaby in your ears and issuing curses in your ear's day in and day out. Not only that, they enter in our unit whenever they want and will steal the smallest article in your home hoping that you might not miss it. They invade your privacy and even if you are hiding pertinent information for only you to have access to it, they have it too. They entered to rob me of anything and everything to drive me into depredation. The thing that they fought me the most for was to send the spirit of infirmity upon me. All of them will have to answer to God, and to mankind because the information is made bare for people to know.

The world we see is just an imitation of another world where enchanters are speaking against mankind on planet earth. Nobody knows that there is another plane that does not touch or meet with the world the natural man inhabits.

COVID19
A Government War against God

Ha! Ha! Ha! Who is going to win? God always
wins, this is not a question that needs an
answer to rather it is to educate those who has
undermine and underestimate my God for an
exceptionally long time and for way to long.

When I got called on the scene, or when the
Lord sent me on the scene, I never realized
that He had chosen me to tackle some
profoundly serious and dark activities taking
place in the belly of hell.   The brain aneurism
that my niece suffered, was my Father's
intention to bring the operation of workers of
iniquity to a halt. Having being in battle with
the dark side that was operating silently in my
life and aiming to give me a brain aneurism,
when I got called on the emergency scene, I
knew exactly where the problem began and
who activated it in hell.
 The devil's children are proud, arrogant,
insolent, and wicked. They came ushering all
types of threats thinking that I might tremble
and turn around and ran. Satan children
specialized in showmanship and he has a
showman waiting to evict a child of God. He
has a showman waiting to eradicate innocent
lives in multitudes. He has a showman waiting
to bring disaster upon disaster on another
innocent man. He has a show man waiting to
represent a child of God to deprive them of

what is rightfully theirs. The showmen are always standing at the door or the front gate. They always act as security guards.

Somehow, the short period that I worked as a security guard, I regarded it as the most crocked profession where people are stripped of their belongings and no one knows what happens to it at the end. Guess what? When I found myself in the lowest pit, and the deepest valleys, people laugh at me. When I was writing poetry upon poetries to express disgust for the accomplishment that brought me no solace, God was laughing, and waiting for this moment. I wrote about achieving a university degree that dug an even greater and deeper pit for me to fall into. I wrote about, rising of condominiums that thrust poverty into a fast-forward mode. I wrote about storage mongers robbing the innocent of goods. I wrote about homelessness and homeless shelters with a false sense of shelter. For whatever reason, I just write out of experience. They were deep bitter lamentations. No one ever read them because they are in storage up to this moment. God reads all of them, and now, He has me addressing them in a totally different light. If anything, I consider myself nothing but the Ambassador in Christ. I have come as a steward serving JESUS. Jesus wants us to serve others, and to be honest with myself, I have been nothing but a servant to another man. And in the eyes of another man, servant brought me much grief through deplorable acts of abuse on my faculty. Today, letting go is painful victory, but the greatest victory is that Jesus is present during it all.

The diagram below gives the individual reader insight on the governance and systemic flow or cycle of how the wicked generate income, and how human lives are manipulated and destroyed in the process.

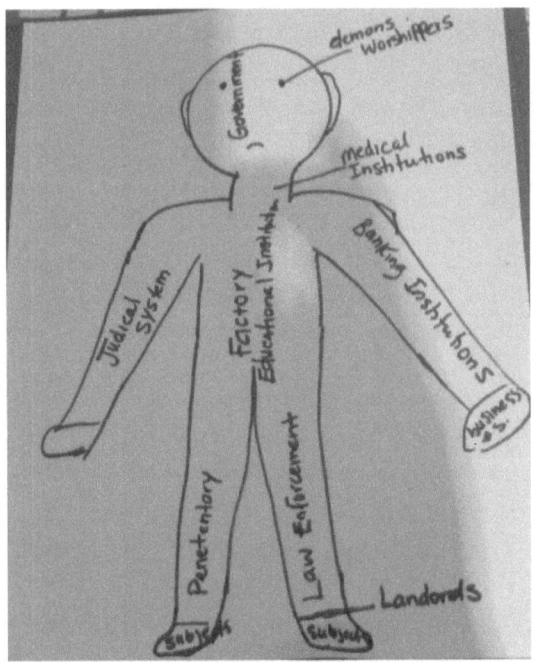

REVOLUTIONARY MOVEMENT
Biblical Revelations and enlightenment by the
word of God

Everything in this world is demonic and
happens and takes place for demonic gains.
Almost every staff washroom has been
transformed into transgender or gender-neutral
washrooms at my workplace. This is an
assault on me as a woman of God and an
insult to the Father that created me. God
created me with perfection and as if some
other being is trying to tell Him he did not know
what He was doing. There is nothing neutral
about me. Despite the rejections, the
oppositions, depressions, depredations, and
whatever else Satanist use to try and put me in
arrested development, God never left my side.
Many rebellions paved the way for us today to
stand against the kingdom of darkness, and
reject all the discrimination, persecutions, and
anything else that causes segregation.
Rebellion revolutionized feminism, but today
there is another type of rebellion formed to
revolutionized genderism and for it to reach a
level or neutralism. Whatever the gimmicks, it
makes no difference to me. It makes a
difference to speak out and let the world know
that there is a satanic rebellion at the root of
every rebellion. In the early beginning of this
trial, I tried to overcome the devil hiding and

remaining confined to a place. They only gained more strength by bringing me to a point of reality. Jesus has won this battle and so have I.

When COVID19 (Corona Virus) is fully accomplished, it is so that people can say that God is Almighty. Many of the white and black magicians have attempted to give the glory to Satan. When the enemy come upon me like a flood, the spirit of God will raise a standard against them. And I tell you the devil never give up and his devilish children never give up. The still fight even after God has emptied their buckets. The efforts to terrorize and terminate is absurd. It even had me thinking that Satan would send a priest to poison a host to kill me faster. It so happened that a recurring vision of people in wheelchairs kept bombarding my field of vision. What I thought it meant to me then that it was part of my vocation until the LORD revealed the true meaning and reason behind the visions. As I learn to co-labor with the Holy Spirit, I became more coherent, and the information the Lord relay become more of a reality that a thought or assumption.

In doing so, I will examine and reveal what the spirit of God has revealed and is about to reveal. **Terminology** plays a key influential role in the organization or institutions. The use of terminology in messages herewith is a culmination of recorded revelations of God, with sets of examples to support evidences. These evidences are containing how the vision of a ladder represents a platform in a stadium for a business model. We are in an age where the ideology of a country is what drives people of a country or nation. We also live in a time where theology has been blotted out from system operations. In this tool you will find an outline that highlight tools and operations.

God told Moses to write down His law's events, testimonies, and ten commandments as a sign for future generations. The sign and wonders of God were should be our template in life for which we build structures to represent God, a platform for us to stand and profess and proclaim the Miracles God performed for the Israelites. And that we should write His laws on the tablet of our hearts. It was so that the same rebellion of the Israelites against Moses would not bring further destruction and calamities on this planet.

While acting as a caregiver for Veronica, the battle was so brutal. This man and woman either possessed her or sent evil spirits to torment her mind. The main purpose that these evil doers wanted to achieve was to break me down physically and mentally. The degree of Psychology that devil worshippers operate under is beyond me.

We hear that evil spirits torment, but the reality is that, evil doers torment. Evil endeavours that are sent against a person is all orchestrated by women and men that are under satanic control. They never work alone, if they are alone is for them to have a meeting with the subject. They come that they might open doors of death and they release something like a skunk so that they can eject themselves into your dreams and inside your unit while you are sleeping.

They will put a man into such deep sleep that they explore, exploit, and leave wicked traces behind to let that person know that they came by and to make their target afraid. And only through the spirit of God and the Wisdom of the Holy Spirit, all the tricks and devises were brought out into the open. God is saying enough is enough.

Suffering at times is immensely and immeasurably intolerable. Darkness always seems to prevail when our hearts are overwhelm with grief. You go to bed wrapped in a tent of darkness. You awoke in the morning in darkness. You cry out over impatience, but what a mighty God we serve.

Oh Lord, I am expressionless, helpless, restless without You. I am powerless like a broken fuse. I am emotional like a leaky faucet. Hurt and pain revisit and refuse to let me forget. In all the interrogation and persecution, I refuse to sign any treaty with witches and wizards. I want the frogs to croak no more, I want the snakes to uncoil and unwound themselves and leave by the Mercy's of God. I do not want to remain volatile and vulnerable to witches and warlocks anymore. They did not want to listen to me, they did not want to listen to God, well it is not by power, not by might but by the power of the Holy Ghost that the truth, which is the word of God shall come to pass. God knows how to break chains and release angels to free man from imprisonments, and He does it the better way, the everlasting way.

A CONTRACT
Signing a Treaty

They answered, "We saw clearly that the LORD was with you; so, we said, "There ought to be a sworn agreement between us' – between us and you. Let us make a treaty with you that you will do us no harm, just as we did not harm you but always treated you well and sent you away peacefully. And now you are blessed by the LORD" Genesis 26:28.

Have you ever heard of the expression that you are signing your life away whenever one is filling out an application or aa contract?

The **psychology** of signing is not clear cut, but what is made more obvious is the contract agreement which is known to be legally binding. We have also been told that what we sign is only a portrait or a template that is open for modification. Thus, goes the reason why a picture tells a thousand words expression circulates. Let me draw an analysis of this paragraph above to explain the predicament that we are all drawn into, and we become the bait and snare of that society. Whenever you are lured into anything it is not by reason or by appearance, but rather by the star that shines above you. The sign that the Lord is with an individual is what draws others to that person. If we analyze this piece further, you notice that the other party want to draw near and get closer because they want to protect their reputation and property.

A contract has nothing to do with friendship. The enemy will not come to develop a friendship. Everything in a contract has to do with autonomy, power over another man that appears to be weaker. If they know that there is an opportunity that you will rise to their challenges, they will forfeit all opportunity and chances that comes your way.

They want to sign a treaty to cover their backbone. They want to sign a treaty, a contract, an agreement not because they are afraid of what their life hold, but rather they are afraid of what they might lose, and in turn gain. We are dealing with liability and assets here, a business method. During the walk on death zones, the enemy trampled my courts, they put barb wire to block my path, they hid sharp nails in my track, they make invocations, they make provocations, they spit, they rant, they shouted, and they fired at me relentlessly. But they always come back and try to shake hands to try and sign a treaty in the spirit realm. Oh! but Jesus! It did not matter the height, the size, or the value of the principal, after Jesus took over my faculty, I just look at their hands in disgust. At times, I would not even acknowledge them.

How can anyone trample and hurt a single, harmless being then come back to suggest a handshake? A regular human being would be ashamed of their behaviors he or she would not even try to come back and apologize while the heat is still on. Satanist like it hot, it is a cooking pot that they must maintain. There are so many things that I am holding back because I have not been able to go back and revisit some of my diaries because they are store away. Right now, I am working with the most recent events. When God gave Moses the ten commandments, we religiously crammed it for the sake of first communion and confirmation. What the Catholic church taught us is so significant and important yet, many of us of did not have a full understanding of the script. When we were young, it was the church duty to educate us with the Word of God. But learning the word without developing curiosity to understand is what it means is ignorance?

Honestly speaking, I still wrestle with this idea and do not know the answer. I did not know the scripture, but I had memorized the Psalm 23 the LORD is my Sheppard. That was the only verse upon which I stood, and man if anyone did me any wrong, I would take the matter right up to the LORD. I watched the LORD brought justice for injustice. I watched the LORD perform miracles in my life. I approached the LORD when I was illiterate in the word, He answered more speedily. We never asked God for big miracles, we always look up to him for little things. Whether it was a habit based on biblical teachings, I do not know.

ECONOMY OF DEATHS

The Legacy

We are living in an era of the economy of
death. We all know a country strives on its
resources, and it determines the transporting of
exports and imports. What we do not know is
how the factory of production and deductions
generate and degenerate human as goods. A
movie projector screen has been spinning,
speeding, and running in an amazingly fast
motion. The common thread that runs through
the projector of my soul is creating a series of a
legacy of family death.

In the similitude of strength God deposited in
my human faculty, it is by that measure that my
characteristics and strength is drawn to
operate and to carry God's torch. I have been
tested and approved by God as a candidate to
carry out God's assignment right through the
darkness and bringing it forth to light.
Oh! How the dark spread its dark sheet over
me that I may not see daylight. Oh! How
wicked foes exploit and explore my vision day
and night. How the wicked enchanter robs me
of my peace. Oh! How wicked enchanters
thought they could deprive me of Heaven's
kiss. Astral projectors enter my sleep and into
my unit. How these wicked men and women
fought to defeat. They harass my life in every
arena with the agenda that we must meet. The
exploit the garbage I dispose in the bin.   They

labor that they might just find a means to drive me into sin. They come with purpose to kill. I would not even dispose of a pin. It does not matter how hard I tried, for them to be effective and for them to affect, we must meet. The fight is to remain on their throne so that we can lose our regular seat.

What do they fight for? Enchanters fight to maintain wealth and property. Enchanters are fighting right now to maintain all the wealth they have stolen throughout generations and up to this generation. What type of battle are we fighting? We are made to believe that the battle is of that of demons. Human beings operate as demons. Devil worshippers have some very clever ways of making things happen from the point of position, to affect and attack a person right inside and outside, using your property and your body. You want to wonder, how it happens. They have operation devices in every area in your room where you most frequented, example in your washroom. They plant things above your head where your fridge is located. The plant things right under your bed and above. The enchanters are silently sitting above you, while the other one sits below.
God is so merciful, but most of all God is the ultimate judge. God sees everything, and I cannot even begin to understand the heightened sense God has bestowed upon me. Whatever God see, He draws my attention to

it. Whatever that displeases God, I find myself looking at the destroyers with contempt and displeasure. Things that once passed as original and regular, I find despicable through the eyes of God.

When my sister's fiancé died a few years ago; somehow, it left me so devastated because of how he died. Joseph's entire system was draining out. He experienced severe bowel for an exceptionally long time to the point that he wobbled while he walked. Whenever, one of my other sisters looked at him, she would say, "there is something wrong with Joseph." The fellow died the most gruesome and grotesque death, that this type of events shall not go unnoticed anymore. When we sit in the audience sit, we do not understand what is written between the lines. Film makers come to make the program to appease and to appeal.

Seeing through the eyes of God is seeing the things that are so painful and inhumane. Travelling and journeying throughout this deserted path and with a feeling of being deserted by everyone is a powerful emotional way of weakening the strength of a person. When I found myself totally hemmed in, without any one to turn to, it made no difference to me whether I lived or died. The reason being is that, if I go back, there was not a single doubt that they would not finish me off. But if I remain in God, I am sure to survive, for God gave me resurrection power and resurrection life that I cannot explain how it came about.

In order that I remain a vessel for God, I have outline everything that God wanted me to reveal. In that very manner I am giving you an anchor as an anchor for survival purposes. The weapons of destructions are both inanimate objects and living things. In the same manner they attack everyone that appeals and appear as cultural oppositions.

When one is vilified, and had their emotions slaughtered, you cannot picture the butcher as a person. Rather we classify this person as a monster. These people may hack away at human flesh, but I will never pollute my life with a lie. Satanist's workstations are located right above and below a victim's bed. There are also others all around you in the North, South, East and West of you. The reason being is that Satanists wants your mind to destroy. The one above your head is manipulating your mind 24/7. The one below you are aiming at your internal organs/intestines and forcing your mind into a mood of needing the washroom. And they continue to do so undetected, undiscovered until you are totally handicapped leading to paralysis.

Satanist workstations are also over the sink where you spend most of your time cooking. They are over the kitchen sink, the face basin and bathtub in the washroom, and even in the laundry room. These are not ordinary human beings; these are assassinator sent to murderer an innocent victim. A victim does not become a scatter brain over night as most people are made to believe. These are very deviant progressive manipulations. Some of the articles or vessels that are being used to achieve such stages are drum beating and loud stomping and banging right over your head. The techniques are so skillful that one can barely hear. You can barely hear is because you are put into a deep sleep. Another of the habit is to move around the room in synchrony with you especially when you go to the washroom. The serpentine sprit or the dragon is being fed right there.

My body developed many types of symptoms, and my system was rapidly deteriorating. And when my body could not retain foods or fluids being fed, I would immediately rush to the washroom until my system became too delicate to hold things in. My unit was experiencing excessive heat throughout the summer and cold during the winter. It was then that the Lord started to pour upon me prophetic number and the acronyms.

HYDRAULICS/After researching the word HYDRAULICS and its meaning -it is described as technology and applied science using engineering, chemistry, and other sciences involving mechanical properties and use of liquids. As a considerably basic level, hydraulics is the liquid counterpart of pneumatics, which concerns gases.

When the Lord revealed the truth, I raised up a standard against the one person I knew was responsible and that is the one above me. He followed me everywhere and rushed to run the water each time. That one was obvious and there was no doubt or maybe about him.

When I went out in a rant and began to call him names, he began with raping me in broad day light. He contaminated the water and put gas down the drain. He contaminated the air releasing gas in the air. Then he began to clog my place and released a stench whenever I am in the bathtub. He contaminated the front door of my apartment every morning with a stench of dead fish; these actions are performed to track me in the night and for other witches and warlocks to torment me during the day. My pubic hair was growing like a wild bush, the more I waxed, the faster it grew. Then I began to realize that the raping would stop until the hair starts shooting out again.

The things these people achieve is so wicked and lengthy. During a visit one night, they filled my right shoe with a dirty liquid, there after chains were attached to my feet in the realm of the spirit. They generate black flies to release in my unit to inject me. When I noticed that vent in the washroom was falling apart, I tried to take it in, but it is one of the outlets for the devil. Things will just fall out of nowhere and break. At times, I can literally feel the anger of something entering in my room. There are vessels planted in the walls without a doubt, and it is right beside my head. Sometimes in the morning, I am awake listening to that thing snoring. While I am typing this, the Holy Spirit is giving me new information, and that is the fellow above me is the one snoring. He seems to have some type of magnetic field drawing information out of me. He came one night and rough me up like a man. He put up something like a dream catcher and warned me not to remove it again. He said quote on quote: **This is the fertility of the house.** People refer to haunting and daunting of unknown experience as devils. Remember human beings are spirits. The reason behind this statement is that, these devil worshippers' keeps fighting to have me come out because they have nothing to work with. Whenever, I go out, one of them must meet me face to face. And whenever I meet with anyone of them, their spirit follows me inside. After each encounter with an old man next door, his spirit enters my apartment and I can literally feel and smell him hanging over my shoulder at the computer. We must remember that these people specialize in things of the spirit realm. They have learned to transform and transmit all types of energy into our homes. The reason why they are called astral projectors is because of their ability to project themselves anywhere and anytime.

When the work of the Lord began to operate in me, my lips could not remain seal forever. Then the Lord began to give me more and more revelations, side by side with ACRONYMS. The Lord gave me a wide scope of numeric prophecy that perhaps have not even been explored or put into terms. Most of what is left unattended would be my fault because my Father did provide much spiritual helpers that explain things to me with such calmness and love. What I must confess is this, at some point fear got in the way and that same fear catapulted the enemy to fight and terrorize me both physically and spiritually. As a victim and witness, I choose to hold nothing back. I have given many explanations and associations to these acronyms as much as possible.

Here are a list of some abbreviations in the very manner the Lord present them/acronyms used by dark men in uniforms, key fundamentals of these properties, and its meanings and functionality are just some of the damages done to innocent victims every day. The acronyms the Lord gave me not just coincide with, but rather describe many of the things presented during the battle with witches. I was key witness and victims to many, and now here to testify about the detrimental impact of what was done to me by the dark side and what they can achieve.

APERS - A person who adopts the appearance or behavior of another, especially in an obvious way. For example, apes, emulators, impersonators, impressionists, mimics. BIPED - An animal that walks on two legs; BIPED – Velocity higher than 1.5 m/s, walking be produced by the chosen actuator, but running is possible. The control law is defined in such a way only the geometric evolution of the BIDEP configuration is controlled, but not the temporal evolution (Cambridge Dictionary). IYU means Organizations, Education, Schools, and other facilities etc. DCNA stands for Data communication network in which your cell phones are hack into. DCNA - Dichloronitroaniline in which your water system is polluted with pesticides. DVW - the DVW is the easiest way to extract data from SAP into Alteryx. If you want to extract data from a business objects system, then checkout the DVW Alteryx (World Wide Web). DWY - A gust or flurry of rain or snow. DWY stands for Driving while yakking and Drug Driving (DUI) (DWI). GRF -Biochemistry, abbreviation for growth hormone-releasing factor: a peptide that is released from the brain and stimulates the pituitary gland to secrete growth hormone (Collins English Dictionary). GRF - stands for Numerology, Chaldean Numerology. The Numerical value of GRF in Chaldean Numerology is 4; Pythagorean Numerology - The Numerical value of GRF in Pythagorean theory. GRF – British English, biochemistry. Abbreviation for growth hormone-releasing factor: a peptide that is released from the brain and stimulates pituitary gland to secrete growth hormone. RCM - Cardiomyopathy Restrictive is heart; RCM - Rehabilitation case Management; RCM - Royal College of Music/RCM - Royal

Canadian Mint produces Canada's circulation coins and collector coins: gold, silver, palladium, and platinum bullion coins [w.w.w].

During all this time of researching the World Wide Web what these abbreviations meant, things were getting deeper and darker. I lost family members during the battle and almost lost a niece during the summer 2019.

One thing I could not pin my finger on was that I had the invisible marks of the stigmata on my hands, feet, my side, and pain on the crown of my head. During the COVID19, the Lord just started to put a spin on other things and brought me new revelations out of the blue. I had a vision of a nail attached to the wall and the part connected to the wall was sort of a rustic dark color. I immediately asked the Lord what this nail is about.

Two days later, the Lord gave me the answer. I woke up in the morning, and the fellow below me was silently nailing my hands and feet. Each time he bangs on the wall, I felt the nail penetrated my body. Then another two days later, the fellow in upstairs followed me to the washroom and he began to silently nail me down. I shouted to him, yes nail me down, nail, nail and I left the washroom. So, there goes the explanation for the stigmata wounds, and how such wounds were being forced into my being by the devil's children.

I began to wonder; how do they achieve such things? The Lord said that they have something representing me, so I thought that it might be my picture. Then later I came up with another idea, another answer that says it is a doll. As soon as I mentioned the event to my sister a few days later, she said, Oh! They have a doll working on you too. I began to laugh the fact that she is giving confirmation about what the Lord showed me.

THE DEATH WISH

Satanists always appear as if by default to meet their victim at the same place each time. These seem as very trivial things that no one pay attention to. They will come about as runners or joggers to send you running for survival. They come as hoarders pushing garbage in a cart as if pushing their belongings around, but one culprit packed the limousine in front of his mansion at nights during the winter. For a person to understand the depth of darkness is having the examples to see and study the despicable manner these people operate. These money mongers outrightly put out old shoes side by side on the sidewalk just as in the day they enter my apartment to wet my shoes with dirty water. They will leave chocolate out on the front doorstep, cigarette boxes, and any other stuff. They put these things outside so that you can see them and develop cravings they also have them on their altar working on a person. They pour out dirty water on the sidewalk waiting for you to walk into. Trivial and petty things win big bucks for them. They leave their body and astral project their wicked self into my space. As I mentioned before, they must have a face to face encounter, and they act so bold that they will literally knock on my door and flee.

These old men and women stink you know. They are willing to take up any persona, pushing grocery carts full of junk, pushing empty baby carriages with junk and it is all for the money. Most time they can drive a victim homeless because their secrets are unheard of. As I finished typed in this section, Jesus just gave me another glimpse of the scroll. I have been frequently meeting men and women wearing a foot brace. Most recently is this guy with a grey and black one. So, this is how after obtaining your property or tamper with your life show, the next step is to but shackles, braces, ropes, chains whatever force they require to restrain a person. So, they chain your feet and to guide your footsteps.

They come walking backwards to catapult your life into backwardness. They slam shut and open doors to throw you out of your home and unto the streets. They open door to lead you into sickness and diseases. They leave doors open with shoes and junk in the doorway to clutter, block your vision. They come by default and thrust their keys in the door at the same time to possess and repossess your apartment. They use shopping carts to block your path, and they trail after you to make you penniless and broke. They asked for information, very subtle details like your internet provider. They spread garbage in your apartment in the spirit realm. Then they get the same provider just to do some stupid thing for you to lose yours. Most things that they do to you in the spiritual realm are carried out in the physical realm.

They monitor and follow you to the bank to control your finances. They curse even with a simple compliment. They make sure that they harass and torment and weary you with threats enough to possess your mind and make you loco. They set off the fire alarm for backup. They point their finger at nothing but that is to lead you were ever they want'to take you, even to the cemetery. They will block the door to block you from meeting your expectations.

They whisper words of contradictions to the word of God in your sleep. People that work in darkness will not hesitate to take chances even after they have been exposed, they want to reverse things. They are superficial and most of what they destroy in another person's life is through artificial means. The come and make serious threats, accusations, blackmail and even issues curse in your ears at nights. They pop up as beggars and beg no one else but you to appeal to pity to give charity so that they can issue curses on vulnerable people. They wait for you on a rock. They wait for you at the three crossroads. They wait for you underneath trees.

The Goliath upstairs pollutes my water with a sticky stench of fish to track me at nights and during the daytime. In that it does not matter how often you bath, the smell remains. That same stench is also what encourages the raping that takes place right under your roof and wherever you go, they go because of the smell on your body. Men and women of God say, it is a demon, but I beg to differ. I had a vision of the fellow sitting topless in a bathtub while the rapist is in action. Other times he is sitting or standing right above my head. Workers of iniquity perform all these wicked activities just to defile a man or woman of God to get them back to sinning against God. In all that raping, my spirit is strongly leading me to some type of solvent, solution, or stimulant of some kind in the water that stimulates the mind, causing me to feel that I am being raped. Clearly, this is not the work of a demon but rather human beings.

My strength is depleting but the Holy Spirit brings me great revival in times of depredations. There is not anyone more dramatic than idol worshippers; they love to stage things, especially when they have been found out.

These people tormented me so much, it is with only Jesus that I maintain my sanity, and to keep from sinning. It is only Jesus that kept me from developing hatred. Wicked, Oh Wicked! Whenever these devil worshippers see me on the streets, they will clear their throats and hack and loud and spit at me. That is to clog my throat to keep silent. The staff members pretended to be hoarse and to pass the curse on to me, and they had me voiceless for a full year, and I could not understand what was going on. Family members were suggesting that I should visit a doctor for it. The Lord pointed out their deviance and treachery to me. They would point at my stomach in mockery and referred to pregnancy to make my stomach balloon.

LIFE AFTER DEATH
Resuscitation verses Resurrection

The term resuscitation is borrowed from the word resurrection. The skillful and clever way that the kingdom of darkness has grown into a huge tree, as the Lord kept showing me in the beginning of this assignment is way too humongous to be simplified. Despite the grandiosity by which such organizations have grown and flourished, nothing is too big for God to tackle. The reason why the enemies massacred my mind and my body was for them to gain some form of advancement against me, thus giving an outlet and clearing the way for them to knock me off the matching line. You know, a person cannot win unless they knock off the opponent whether it is by plotting the death of that person or by laying stumbling blocks in the way.

Fighting against me meant that they were fighting against God. I made daily declarations reinforcing and reminding these slayers that they were fighting against God. The statement meant nothing to them for the only thing they beheld was the image of me as another regular person. You see, the ability they have gained and the weapons of destructions they used for decades were how strength were build and it was how they carry out wiping out nations in secrecy.

You see, they use the Scripture, but they do not follow the instructions lay down by God. You see, they use the scripture to measure and track time, and this is how therefore they use the time clock, a watch, or any method of time to keep a record of how God operates. However, that time piece is useless to them without a man of woman of God to follow around and prey upon. You see, a man or woman of God is built and design to carryout God's plan and purpose.

When we do not know God, we do not know who we are. We do not know the plan and purpose that God has set in place that will lead and guide us to the walking the line of Divinity. Without God, Satanist draw other lines to divert and deviate our path and our thoughts.

The first thing God made me to understand when I got reborn was the fact that I did not have an identity. After giving my life to Christ, I developed a new self- confidence, one that give me a new self-image. But it was while finding myself in the unit of death, that I began to look in the mirror and noticed that my eyes were the eyes of God. Somehow, I was looking into the eyes of JESUS. I am not just saying this folk it is a fact, perhaps I had grown cocky, or so I thought. But it is during this very hour and period the plan and purpose of God was recovered. It is in this very place that very unit of death that my heart was reshaped, and my body recalibrated to generate the embodiment of a Christ-like body. What I did not know was that all along God, the Great Potter was reshaping and remolding my body. God the Great Autor was re writing the script of my life that the devil's children had trampled upon mashing up my flesh like cornfields. You see, they had been working for a long time in secret you see.

The devil works in succession and quite slowly in some cases, so that no one will suspect foul play. My tolerance for the adversities causes by adversaries reached new level of intolerance. Everything that I experienced while under the experiment of devil worshipper though out brough to a standpoint to sound my alarm bell to call an emergency alert. Many of the vessels they use are explored in other works, the use of the fire alarm, the bell, the drum, monitoring devices, in some cases I explored the alarm bell, the sensor, and much more.

Remember, Satanist cannot and will never walk around without wearing a mask. These masqueraders come with a mile. These masqueraders using high professional titles and wearing pretty uniforms. These masqueraders know and loves to give compliments. These masqueraders love to shake hands to steal you anointing and virtues. Remember that they are the ones who come up with shaking hands and looking them in the eyes during an interview. I have looked into multiple eyes and never got the job. These masqueraders are your most intimate neighbors because they are on your left, on your right and above and below. These masqueraders pretend to be your best friend. Remember when you go to the North, you meet them by default. When you go to the south you meet them by default, when you go to the East, you meet them by default. And when you go to the West there they are. They have orchestrated a plan, a way of following your footsteps. This is an indication meaning, they have gotten access to your shoes, your property somehow. In case you miss the point, it has been laid bare as a repetition for God's servants to know, see and understanding surrounding afflictions that threatens one's livelihood.

Oh! Eternal Truth – Make me an instrument of Your love. To be as shrewd as a serpent and as gentle as a dove. I am languishing in the flames of darkness. Let your presence dispel falsity. Oh! Eternal Truth. Open my lips to dispel of unforetold reality this day. I empty my vessel before You Lord to be purified. I have been robbed and stripped undignified. Let Your Holy fire ravage and burn the wild weeds within. Oh! Eternal Truth, my heart bleeds. Before You I cry and plead. In Your Holy presence, angels raise their shields. My JESUS, my LORD, and my GOD. Oh! Eternal

Truth. Train me in all manner to use Your sword. Before You I yield. Help my wounds heal. So, I may no longer remain the same man the sword once wields. I want to wield that sword.

Symbolism – Lord, let this cup pass. Do not whip my love. My eyes drink the Blood that flows from Your wounded heart. I present my body bruised and bath in ashes in a loin cloth. The wrath and the lashes by our brothers and sisters, have me fleeing for cover. I held in my hand a blood-soaked handkerchief. It is unjustifiable what my lips will not utter. Bound by paralytic fear. Oh! King of justice who undo injustices. JESUS, my JESUS. You are the Prince of Peace. I want to run. I am caught in the Armageddon. Oh! The Autumn daffodils bloom. Judge of all men who declared my doom, come.

Father, I offer my prayer to You. I long to hear You say that You love me. It is my desire that through my confessions, oppressions, depressions, and professions that souls will be lifted to heaven. Lord, I call your name soiling my blanket with tears. Let my distress exhume dead spirits hidden in our midst. Lift your hands oh Lord. Let conversion of souls resurrected dead flesh. I am lifting and beholding the cross in fantasy to get to heaven. I call unto the Lord in great ecstasy of the Holy Spirit. Make haste and make my dreams a reality. Let me stand

no more in false hope overlooking the bay.
Take my empty hands in thine, I pray. I am the
branch; you are the Vine. You are truly Divine.

July 19, 2019 My sister Sandy is asking me to
look after my niece for her. A pair of hands
were reaching out with a bouquet of purple
flowers. July 22, 2019 a cop or a pilot took a
suitcase and left. July 27, 2019, I had a vision
of a factory burning and someone who looked
like OW fainted. July 27, 2020, I had a vision of
a wooden cross, and then multiple other
crosses started to surface in all types of colors.
July 30, 2020, I had a vision of a creature rising
from the water. August 31, 2019, I had another
vision of a creature rising out of the water.

Broken Wings – I am still flying on broken
wings. I turn into a butterfly, then into a moth. I
lay down at the Valley of Succoth. The life I
live does not correspond with the song that I
sing. I am just a sling shot away. They tell me
stories to throw me in disarray. Dragons
comes along spitting fire. I am still flying on
broken wings. Blessed with Divine unique
ability. I am standing on a stool of instability.
The competitor comes in sequence. I no
longer try to make sense out of nonsense. I
lay down at the Valley of Succoth. There I was
discovered by the Divine Savior.

The age of the valley is upon us. In the Valley
of Aven, the word of the LORD says, *I will send*

a fire upon the house of Hazael, and it shall devour the strong hold of Ben-hadad. I will break the gate bar of Damascus and cut off the inhabitants in the Valley of Aven Amos1:4-5. For the day of the Lord is near in the valley of Decision. The sun and the moon are darkened, and the stars withdraw their shining Joel 3:14. Let the nations stir themselves up and come to the valley of Jehoshaphat. For there I will come to judge Joel 3:12. The valley of Jezreel, Then Jehu went to Jezreel. When Jezebel head about it, she puts on eye makeup, arranged her hair, and looked out of a window. As Jehu entered the gate, she asked, have you come in peace you zimri, you murderer of your master? He looked up at the window and called out. "Who is on my side?" "Who?" Two or three Eunuchs looked down at him. Throw her down! Jehu said. So, they threw her down, and some of her blood splattered the wall and the horses as they trampled her underfoot.

The things that is most engrained is the fact that the forger thrust above me was sent to come and shift my perspective about God. He has indeed shifted my entire spiritual framework. In order that God would accomplish His plan and purpose for my life God brough many unexpected changes. *Then I took even my staff Beauty and cut it asunder that I might break my covenant which I had made with the people Zechariah 12:9.*

God severed all ties that I had with another human being. In the isolation, my family members did not know what I was going through, nor did they hear from me. Then God even went further to remove the people that I would rely on for help and share God's secrets with them. Essentially, the people that were the driving force pushing the darkness, they were people that I trusted. God made it so easy that they took it up on their own to banish me from the church and they were ultimately fighting to drive me off my workplace entirely. There were several attempts to fire me on the job just because men of Satan thought that by getting rid of me, they will have me in a powerless state so as not to ever see the fulfilment of God's prophecy come to pass. With my God beside me, I fought, I wage war against them.

Then I cut asunder my other staff Bands, that I might break the brotherhood between Judah and Israel Zechariah 12:14.

While this is not a sound of victory for me but to God, I find myself going through a different type of groaning. The whole battle taught me a type of reality. These men living below and above me have shifted me to a new altitude. While the voice of injustices still rings. The gripping truth of 400 years in battle still echoes.

My Father has had enough of the puppet master's show.

The Lord made His promise good, He said after joy comes sorrow. *Rejoice Zebulun in your going out, and you Issachar in your tents. They will summon people to the mountain. And there offer the sacrifices of the righteous. They will feast on the abundance of the seas, on the treasures hidden in the sand"* Deuteronomy 33:19.

I cry when nobody knows why I cry. I laugh when nobody knows why I laugh. I lick my tears like ice-cream. I find warmth in heaven's beam. I work in a kingdom of adversity. I work understanding the world of reality to be a place to pity. I fought to shake dirt off my skin. The war is severe dragging with its famine. Today my soul melts like burning flax. Memories tears me to pieces like an axe. Oh, Messiah help me sing. Oh Lord of lords, King of kings. You entered my will and emotions to break down walls of adversity. To see what I see, feeling what I feel. With a heavy heart I pass through the fire. I cut through barb wire and trample the mire. Oh Messiah, Messiah, Messiah. There is a hit woman on a rock near three trees. Oh! Let her flee. The enemy circle me like bees. Oh, keeper of hidden silencer. Waiting to pull the trigger at the three crossroads. Oh, assassinators will groan like toads. They have expanded their repertoire. Oh! wicked

Oh! Death where is thy sting. Oh, how I have become hot commodity for Satan's children.

Victimization makes a lousy student out of a human being. Experience is a brutal instructor using grueling force in trainings. In our lifetime we will and must counter both of such characters that comes either to shape or shade our identities.   It is with such encounter that human development starts to take shape. Psychological teachings of organizations are tragically and statically impels monuments of tragedies to bring a man to an arrested development stage of worthlessness. Teacher, instructors, facilitators, tells us about moto and model skills. I like to put it that way because human like a vehicle going on a test drive. We can either fail or pass the test drive. My experience behind the wheels of survival… were determinant and detriments. Where do we go from here? The most recent line most used for me "I am going to fight my own battles" meaning be careful who I but heads with.   Workers of iniquity once told me that they thought that I was one of them. Jesus has not call me to match on that line of duty.

The beginning of summer school vacation is a season in time where many students and school staff gravitate towards. As for me a temporary staff, it has been a nightmarish time year after year. Spending months at home without an income has been a cyclone of financial disruptions. More importantly, mentioning the disparity of the political laws and bylaws of this nation is more bias and crippling in all of it ways and in all humanity. The policies and politics are loaded guns.

Imagine paying into unemployment and when the time comes, laws, claws, loopholes and whatever stinking gook or junk that Ontario government has been sending my ways has been way overloaded. The tore the flesh in my arms to bring my arms down. I tolerated the funk and the junk way too long. Sinking deep into the grassroots of systemic discrimination, prejudice, racism, the impeachment on laws and claws had gripe me long enough. The catalyst for death toils, homelessness, crimes, are in scripted into laws and statutes of this nation. Describing times of destitution and its destructive force against my physical, emotional, and spiritual wellbeing is nerve wrenching. Speaking of demonic habitation, society thinks it is taboo, wait until they hear what I have to say.

We knew no other god(s) but JESUS. But the other gods are hidden among us as figurines, good luck charms, and jewelry. We may not directly bow to them nor will we ever serve them. Yet we dust them and shine them and build glass homes or cabinets for them. What struct me when entering a Chinese or Indian store was the pressure from store owners and clerks that moved me to purchase things that I never intended to spend on nor was it needed. Spending a large part of my income which should have been my savings in China town, and Indian discount stores my life ebbed away as financial disaster hem me in a dark cave. There was a time in my life when I was lost in translation.

Looking at evil doers and knowing the degree of afflictions they are putting me through along with my family and what evil the perform on others, I find it rather revolting. Opening doors for me as a generous gesture is sickening, and I want to tell it to their faces and to the world. They are killing, afflicting, and trafficking human beings by the second. Satanists is not messing with my family one bit, not anymore. Not if my Jesus have me on the training ground. And they are mad. everyone in this season is experiencing heat rising out of the underworld. They want us to believe that it is a climate change. To the very rising of condominiums to skyscrapers or sky risers, God's law is against it. Think about what god says about the tower of babel.

This is not a joke. When the truth is addressed, people think that one is crazy and stupid. In that moment of truth is intellectualism is showcased. With a string of evidence, a string of vicious attacks, a string of vicious acts dominating and destroying lives are hidden in the dust. They are unraveling and un-bended rules that apply to concretize appearances are microscopic. It is wedged, embedded, deep in hard rocky soil and it is as laborious as discovering relics. People are dying and the author of death sits on his throne while his tyrants destroy. We have been made to believe that we have no control of death, I beg to differ. The standard of this world are platoons and platforms where Satanists match and leave their marks. And each department keeps a logbook with a rubric of the number of men slain. They leave footprints, fingerprints, tombstones, graves, reaves, corpse and what more? What more LORD?

Drawbacks are building blocks raised high to block our landscapes, and workers of iniquity are imbeciles, building monuments of death through insincere relationships, immaturity, fictitious in personalities. They will keep spreading propaganda and lies. Thinking without reasoning, unreliable witnesses…social intellects and with other defects. They use flattery to chaperone and tailgate presume ignorant individuals. when they went after

Jesus, they were bent on crucifying him even though all the evidences against him were orchestrated and planted just to trap him. It was made known to the public spectators that this man is innocent, but everyone gathered with one accord to go against Jesus. The bible record and the evidence of Jesus' innocence, and the evidence of Jesus' innocence still stands today.one of the most resounding statement that Jesus made was, they will persecute you for my sake. When Jesus made that statement, it never tells us what to prepare for, but composing and writing this piece comprise of graphic sketches of the underlayers of death by injustices, and how judgement is passed for crimes and punishments. Writing and working behind the scenes makes character sketches easier to draw. Not being a witness is more often as safer stance to take. But without and over seer, someone to relate and correlates information, oversights are never reviewed and corrected. Whatever piece he is composing another man is compromising what it comprises.

In the face of adversity, a hand ticks waiting for the alarm bell to sound off. Church steeple reduced as fire rages. It is the sign of beast ages. They come to kill and destroy. The world bare extraordinarily little record of whom Satan has employed. Destruction is upon our land. Robbers lying wait, band of robbers.

Exterminators position to shoot right into your shoes. In that manner, they may control your where abouts. Walking the streets of Toronto is more deadly than walking on landmines or walking a battle line. It is all systematically programmed that a certain ratio, type, prototype, and genetically coded beings must die prematurely. All the tramps that sedated, seduced, and secluded me just to force me into submission will eventually answer to my God. A person is useless to Satan unless one is dead, and their soul transported to hell.

The very act of kindness such as opening and holding a door open is a a trap for one to enter a pathway of death leading to hell. Even a handshake in an interview is a set up. My abode is a coven. They set traps all around to ensnare me and think that people that have blank expressions are all blindfolded still. The ammunition is being loaded and reloaded in a blank stare in the heavens. I have previously mentioned many aspects of strategically applied mechanisms.

They think that I am still playing patter cake, patter cake, bake my bread. They are still trying to determine how big a loaf that should be in my fridge. It has been a constant struggle keeping bread on my shelf. Not knowing that elves was hiding in my cupboard, I kept feeding them. Even trying to starve the devil is an exchange because of constant game change. Somehow, they believe that I am lost in transition. Oh! How they have solicited God's goodness and mercy.

I am no longer in the game, but they are so busy creating movies, they refuse to accept that the opponent is now a victor. The rhetoric, to mislead individuals so that their preys are gullible and entrapped. They ought to know by now that there is a game change. In as much as evil doers are game changers, the never expected the opponent to switch gear on them. The reason for the miscalculation is because they like to tailgate the prey. Living this life and relying on others to determine our worth and to define whatever information we are given is to live in full ambiguity.

Today June 6, 2020, the fellow pollutes the air and contaminate the water with poop stench. It is not my poop that he uses anymore because I have not used the toilet in over two years. So, it stands to reason that he prepared a portion with his own poop to throw down at me. I said nothing but took it to social media next day.

They will pose as cops to make corpses out of Christians. Many powerful trees bend their backs to COVID19. Bending their backs to the control team. They occupy seats on buses to command people to conform. This is not the norm. They have fast forwarded the revelation of God. The wicked refuse to adhere. Fighting

that I may fall under subjection to Satan.
Thinking that I would die when public
washrooms got banned. God strengthened me
so that I can endure for a whole week. Is it not
enough that they have wearied me? Then they
must weary my God too. I come to bring out all
that is true. I come that all flesh may be silent.
I come in the name of JESUS, God of love that
is kind and patient. I come in the name of the
LORD. I come stretching His measuring rod.
There comes a time when an apology
becomes an offense. What real man or
woman would eve think that I would sell my
JESUS for six pence. The blood of JESUS, let
it rise. Let it touch some lives.

June 9, 2020 It has been six or seven day
straight since I last use the washroom.
I left the apartment to go and use the
washroom somewhere. Whenever I go out to
use the washroom, it is a waging war against
human devils. When I return to the building,
the black woman with her black cat opened her
door all the way and she was hiding behind the
curtain. I stood on the doorstep calling
repentance. Just when I turn my camera off
and push my key in the door to enter, the
fellow from above me came out like a rabbit out
of a borrow. Then another fellow that played
me and plagued me in the beginning came out
like the hare out of it hole and they are ready
for marathon to see who can run me down
faster. It is how they operate you know. They

will ambush the opponent and strike in the spirit realm. The one above was just too anxious to fire his weapon for it had not been his intension that he be seen. JESUS is LORD. They are aware that they are no longer mysteries to me, so they waste no time to shoot.

Suddenly, these men and women that present themselves with doctorates, and so on, began to meet with me in unexpected places. What kind of doctor are they? Doctor Kill! They are no longer holding the agenda upon which they strive to accomplish.

When I went about and purchase an expensive camera, I never imagined or anticipated that I would ever walk with a video camera across Toronto, calling for repentance. This is a clear-cut sign that without God a video camera is useless. The LORD had me shift my perspective on the way I look at things. The LORD has certainly position me among a list or group of workers of iniquity as a force representing God. It is with that same purpose that those who labor to kill me every day watch the power of God unfolds.

Therefore, you Israelites, I will judge each of you accordingly to your own ways declares the LORD. Repent! Turn away from all your offenses; then sin will not be your downfall.

Rid yourselves of all the offenses you have committed, and get a new heart and a new spirit, why will you die, people of Israel? For I take no pleasure in the death of anyone, declares the Sovereign LORD. Repent and live! Ezekiel 19:30-32.

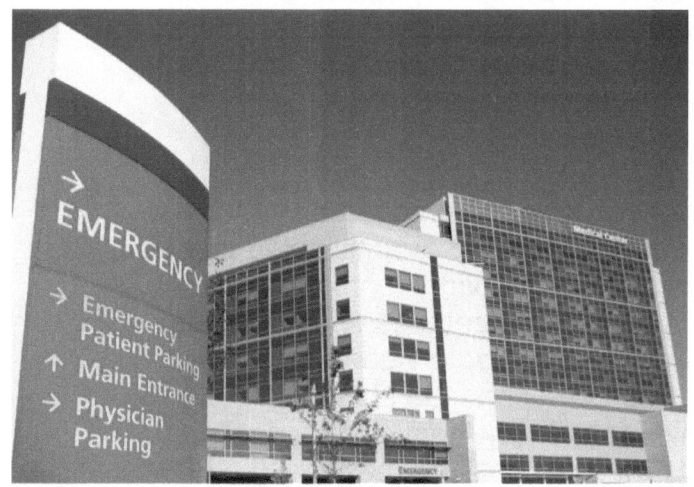

www.ingramcontent.com/pod-product-compliance
Lightning Source LLC
Chambersburg PA
CBHW030947240526
45463CB00016B/2059